THE SPACE WE HOLD, THE SPACE WE NEED

A Short Narrative into the Soul of Nursing

Angela Swanson, MSN, RN

The Space We Hold, The Space We Need

Copyright © 2025 by Angela Swanson, MSN, RN.

MILTON & HUGO L.L.C.
4407 Park Ave., Suite 5
Union City, NJ 07087, USA

Website: *www. miltonandhugo.com*
Hotline: *1- 888-778-0033*
Email: *info@miltonandhugo.com*

Ordering Information:
Quantity sales. Special discounts are granted to corporations, associations, and other organizations. For more information on these discounts, please reach out to the publisher using the contact information provided above.

Library of Congress Control Number: 2025917288
ISBN-13:   979-8-89285-617-1   [Paperback Edition]
                  979-8-89285-629-4   [Hardback Edition]
                  979-8-89285-616-4   [Digital Edition]

Rev. date: 07/22/2025

PREFACE

To Gavin and Olivia—

You are the truest reasons I ever learned to hold space.

It was your small hands, your bedtime stories, your soccer games and football games I missed while caring for strangers. It was your quiet patience while I slipped through the door hours late, still wearing the day's weight in my eyes. It was your laughter echoing down the hallway that reminded me there was still joy waiting for me outside the hospital walls. You are the reason I kept showing up for others -- and the reason I kept coming home.

Thank you for loving me through every missed dinner, every exhausted hug, every shift that left me hollow and distant. You gave me grace when I had none left for myself. You helped me become a mother and a nurse in tandem -- and you never made me choose between the two. I hold space in this world because you taught me how to hold love in its most powerful form.

To my fellow nurses—

This book is for the ones who know.

For the ones who sit silently in supply closets and cry between codes. For those who know what it means to bear witness without words. For the nurses who tape their shoes, offer up their last caffeine tablet, cover shifts when their bones ache, and still manage to ask, "Are you okay?"

You are the ones who understand that medicine doesn't always save, that healing sometimes looks like presence, and that showing up -- fully human, fully exhausted, fully determined -- is a sacred act. You are not just the backbone of healthcare. You are the soul.

This space is for you. You've held it for everyone else. Let this book hold it for you.

To the friends and family who love us—

Thank you for being our soft landing.

Thank you for the texts we never answered, the calls you kept making anyway, the understanding that sometimes silence means "I can't talk about it yet." You have stood by us without needing the details, loved us without needing the explanation, and given us the room to unravel without fear of being unworthy.

You loved us through our numbness, through our short answers and our long disappearances. You saw the toll this work took and never asked us to be anything other than human. You reminded us who we were beyond the badge—and you gave us permission to come back to ourselves.

This is your dedication, too.

INTRODUCTION

The First Time I Held Space

I was a baby nurse -- fresh off orientation, still second-guessing every step, and crying in the supply closet more days than not. I thought I understood what nursing would be. I had passed exams, learned to hang fluids, and practiced inserting IVs on mannequins until my hands moved on autopilot. But none of that prepared me for this—for the way the air could shift when life was slipping away. For the silence that sometimes followed screaming. For the moment I realized I wasn't just there to heal—I was there to hold.

It was early in my career, on an ortho-neuro floor -- a place where people could be talking and laughing at breakfast and gone by dinnertime. That day, I was assigned a new patient being transferred from the ER. She was in her 40s -- younger than my mother. On vacation when it happened. A massive hemorrhagic stroke. The kind that offered no recovery, only waiting.

No one teaches you how to walk into that room. No one prepares you for the moment you realize your job is not to make someone better -- but to make their death less alone.

I stood at the doorway and hesitated. My hands shook. My stomach clenched. She was unconscious, but her presence filled the room. There was still so much of her there, and I didn't know how to meet that with anything but fear.

The hospitalist came in shortly after. He rattled off her prognosis like he was reading from a grocery list -- monotone, impersonal, already halfway out the door. There was no softness. No pause. No acknowledgment of who she had been. I felt heat rise in my chest. I challenged him. I didn't plan to -- the words just came. I said she wasn't just a diagnosis. She was someone's mother. Someone's wife. Someone's everything. And she deserved to be seen.

Later, her family arrived. They got there just in time. She passed with her husband holding one hand and me holding the other. When it was over, he hugged me. He didn't thank me for saving her. He thanked me for sitting with her. For staying. For treating her like she mattered, even in her final hours.

That moment shaped me.

That was the first time I understood what it meant to hold space. Not in the abstract, but in the raw, aching, human way. To sit beside someone when nothing can be fixed. To be a witness to both the dignity and the devastation. To carry the weight of what it means to stay present when every part of you wants to run.

Over time, I learned to carry those moments like sacred stones in my pocket. Quiet markers of where I had been and who I had become. I stopped trying to numb them. I let them shape me.

I've collected so many stories since then -- some brutal, some beautiful. Each one stitched a little deeper into who I am. Every nurse has them -- a gallery of invisible memories. We don't always speak them aloud, but we never forget.

This book is a short narrative into the soul of nursing. A glimpse into the rooms, the hallways, the supply closets, and the in-between spaces where the real work happens -- not just the healing, but the holding.

These pages are for the nurses who have lived it, and for the people who love us enough to try and understand.

1

The Unseen Cost

You can't chart the weight we carry.

There's no drop-down menu for the moment your patient asks, "Am I dying?"

No checkbox for the times you held your bladder for eight hours because no one could cover you for a break. No field in the EMR to log the tears you swallowed after zipping a body bag shut.

People see the scrubs. The badge. The stethoscope. They might even see skill, efficiency, maybe compassion if they're paying attention. But they don't see the unraveling that happens behind the supply room door. They don't see the toll this work takes on your body, your spirit, your family.

They don't see you at the end of a shift, sitting in your car in the parking lot, frozen, gripping the steering wheel, knowing that once you let go -- once you exhale – it'll all come pouring out.

They don't know what it's like to drive home in silence, windows down, music off, just trying to remember how to feel human again. You pull into your driveway and sit there, still in your scrubs, wondering if you have the energy to walk inside and pretend you didn't just hold someone's child as they died.

There's an invisible cost to being a nurse.

It's not just exhaustion -- though that alone can be crushing.
It's the emotional contortions we perform.
The need to switch from comforting a grieving family to joking with a pediatric patient in five minutes flat.
The husband who brings flowers to his wife's bedside, knowing it's the last bouquet.
The woman who grips your hand and begs you not to let her die alone.

The things we carry home aren't always the ones we can talk about. Sometimes, they're not even the ones we fully understand. They live in our bodies, our sleep, our silence.

I remember a teenager who coded right in front of us. One minute she was laughing -- alive -- and the next, we were running. Tubes. Hands. Shouts. Silence.

There are some deaths you carry like bruises. You can't show them to anyone, but they're always there.
That one never left me.

And the stroke patient -- she was my mother's age. She never got the chance to speak. I advocated for her when no one else did. Pushed back against the kind of detachment that turns patients into problems to be solved. She died peacefully, but I still remember how her husband hugged me and thanked me not for saving her -- but for seeing her.

You become the keeper of stories too heavy for daylight conversation.

The quiet witness to grief, grace, and sometimes unimaginable loss.

So we patch ourselves together in small ways.

A coffee before shift.
A nurse friend who meets your tired eyes and just nods.
A playlist you cry to when the house is finally quiet.
Shoes that don't hurt your feet.
Routines you create to survive.

And still -- we show up.

Because behind the heartbreak is something else, too.
The reason we stay.

The moment someone looks at you like you're their lifeline.
The way a man softens when you gently place a blanket over his shoulders.
The whispered thank you that echoes even after the room is empty.

The unseen cost is real.

But so is the love.

And for many of us, that's enough to come back -- again and again -- to
the space we hold.

Chapter

2

Every Death is Memorable

People always ask, "How do you do it?"

They mean, how do you survive being around so much death?
They think it becomes routine. That we get used to it.
But we don't.

You never get used to watching someone take their last breath.
Not when it's a teenager who coded in front of you.
Not when it's a newborn you swaddle, knowing the blanket will outlive
the baby.
Not when it's someone who reminds you of your own family -- your
grandmother, your father, your child.

Every death is memorable.
Not because of how someone died -- but because of who they were.
Because of what they left behind, or what they finally let go of.

Some go quietly, like a candle snuffed out without warning.
Others rage and tremble until the last second.
Some families fall apart in grief.
Some somehow fall back together.

There was a homeless Vietnam veteran I'll never forget. He was at the end of his life -- and he knew it. He had no visitors, no requests. But he had once been someone. I could feel that.

The trauma was etched into his movements. His voice was soft but sharp.

I stayed with him as he died. I didn't have a reason beyond: no one else would.

And I remember how the light hit his face just as his breath faded. It was simple. Dignified. Like the world paused for him.

There was a husband who sang to his wife as she slipped away.

A daughter who whispered, "I forgive you" through tears and oxygen masks.

A woman who looked just like my grandmother -- she let me brush her hair the night before she passed. "This makes me feel like I matter," she whispered. That moment -- more than any code or procedure -- is what stuck.

The small human things we do before the body lets go.

And then there are the deaths that come like earthquakes.

A teenager once coded in front of us. One minute she was laughing, the next we were running. Compressions.

Meds. Shouting. Silence.

We did everything. It wasn't enough.

There's a special kind of grief when someone dies who hasn't had a chance to live yet.

You carry that one like a bruise that never fades.

You stop thinking of "time" as something guaranteed.

Some deaths are peaceful. Others are unbearable.

But all of them leave something behind.

A phrase. A sound. A feeling you can't shake.

There was a young woman I cared for -- my age, with cancer. We talked in stolen moments between scans and nausea. She had two kids. She knew what was coming. And she carried that knowing with grace I still can't comprehend.

She didn't ask me to save her.
She asked me to remember her.
And I do.

Every death teaches us something we didn't want to learn.

We become carriers of last words.

Holders of final breaths.
Witnesses to goodbyes that no one else saw.

We tuck these people away in our minds like photographs that never fade.
We remember the face. The sound. The stillness after.

We keep a gallery of them in our hearts.
Not because we can't let go -- but because we shouldn't.

Every death is memorable.

Because every life meant something.

Chapter

3

We Laugh So We Don't Cry

There's a kind of laughter that echoes down hospital halls -- sharp, too loud, sometimes completely out of place.
It cuts through the sound of monitors, overhead calls, and quiet despair like a jolt to the chest.

It's not unprofessional. It's necessary.

We laugh because if we didn't, we'd break.

I worked in a trauma hospital in the PACU -- the kind of place where chaos was a constant. Emergencies didn't happen in waves; they happened all at once. Staffing was always short. Tension was always high. But somehow, we kept each other upright. And we laughed.
God, we laughed.

There was an anesthesiologist we all adored.
He cracked jokes right up until the patient was out cold. Not cheap ones -- smart, cutting, perfectly timed humor that disarmed everyone in the room. He could walk into a disaster and make people breathe again. He once said to me, "You've gotta learn to be funny in a fire. It's the only way you can stand the heat."

And he was right.

Laughter wasn't the opposite of pain -- it was the release valve.
It let some of the pressure out before it tore us open.

I remember one day during a particularly brutal shift, a patient woke up from anesthesia and burst into a full karaoke performance. I mean full-on, eyes closed, hand motions, slurred lyrics and all. We were exhausted. Emotionally wrung out. But in that moment, we lost it -- full-body laughter. That kind of laugh that starts in your ribs and ends in tears.

And then there was the code where someone farted during compressions.

We were elbow-deep in trauma and panic, but that sound snapped the tension like a rubber band. For a second, we were human again. We let ourselves laugh -- not because it was funny, but because the grief was about to swallow us whole and the only other option was to scream.

People on the outside might think we're insensitive.

But we're not.
We just learned that grief sits too heavy in silence.
So we fill the cracks with sound.

Laughter became a way to say: I'm still here.
You're still here.
We made it through another one.

Because sometimes, we come home and stare at a wall.
We cry in the shower.
We sit in our cars long after the engine's off, trying to remember how to feel something other than numb.
But for a few moments on the floor -- in a hallway, a breakroom, a shared glance -- we laugh.
And in that moment, we breathe.

There's a saying: Laughter is medicine.
But in nursing, it's more than that.
It's CPR for the soul.

It's how we keep going.
We laugh so we don't cry.
And sometimes, we do both at the same time.

Chapter

4

Not Just a Nurse

There's a phrase we hear far too often:
"I know you're just a nurse, but..."

It's usually followed by a question they think we're not qualified to answer -- or a request they assume we'll carry out without question. It's always delivered with that same tone.
Condescending. Casual. Dismissive.

As if being a nurse is somehow a lesser form of being.

I remember finishing my master's program -- a mountain of work. Night shifts, research papers, clinical hours, parenting, and pushing myself through every ounce of self-doubt. When I finally submitted my final paper, I was proud. I told one of the trauma surgeons I worked with that it had ended up being thirty-eight pages.

He raised an eyebrow and smirked.

"How many of those pages had pictures?"

I forced a laugh. Said, "None. I'm a nurse. Not a doctor."

He nodded. Not unkindly. But it stayed with me. Because even in a moment of pride, even among colleagues, I wasn't seen as equal. I was something adjacent. Something helpful. Supportive. But not central.

That mindset is everywhere.

People don't realize how much we know -- or how we know it.

They think it all comes from textbooks. But a lot of it comes from time. From being present. From the kind of noticing that doesn't fit neatly on a resume.

We hear the change in a patient's voice before the monitors sound.
We see the subtle shift in skin tone that tells us something's coming.
We watch family dynamics unfold and know, within minutes, who's going to fall apart.
We catch missed orders, miswritten meds, vitals that don't look right.
And we advocate. Fiercely. Quietly. Constantly.

Because we know what's at stake.

Being "just" a nurse means you know how to lead without needing credit.
It means you learn how to work the system -- not to cheat it, but to protect people from it.
It means showing up with a thousand layers of knowledge no one sees, and still being the one who holds the hand when things fall apart.

And here's what they don't say out loud:
We are the ones patients trust the most.
Not because we have the title.
But because we've been there -- at the bedside, in the moment, with the weight of it all on our shoulders.

There is no "just" in what we do.

We are not assistants to someone else's brilliance.

We are brilliant in our own right.

We are not lesser.
We are essential.

So the next time someone says, "Just a nurse," I hope they hear how absurd that sounds.

Because what we do?
It saves lives.
It heals families.
It holds this broken system together.

We are nurses.

And there is nothing "just" about that.

Chapter

5

Can I Brush Your Hair

Sometimes it's not the lifesaving interventions that matter most.
Sometimes healing begins with a simple question:
"Can I brush your hair?"

I remember the elderly woman clearly.
She reminded me so much of my grandmother -- her wit still sharp, her eyes still searching, even as her body gave out.
She had been through it all. Multiple admissions, tests, strangers waking her up at 2 a.m. to poke and prod.
She didn't ask for much.

But I could tell -- she felt forgotten.
Her hair was matted. Her gown was wrinkled. Her spirit was dim.
She didn't complain. She didn't need to.
I saw it in the way she avoided mirrors. The way she looked past people instead of at them.

So I offered her something small.
Something human.
"Would you like me to brush your hair?"

At first, she hesitated -- as if the kindness startled her.

As if she wasn't sure if she was allowed to receive care that wasn't tied to a diagnosis.

But then she nodded. Softly. Almost shy.

I found a comb in the drawer. I pulled a chair close.
And I began brushing, slow and gentle, working through the knots with more care than I could put into words.

We didn't talk much.
But her eyes softened. Her shoulders dropped. Her breathing deepened.

"This makes me feel like I matter again," she whispered.

That moment -- that quiet, ordinary moment -- stayed with me.

Because nurses are trained to assess, to intervene, to stabilize.
We're taught to watch the numbers. Hit the metrics. Document the data.

But there's another kind of medicine.
The kind that lives in the smallest acts.
A warm blanket. A hand to hold. Lotion rubbed into cracked feet.
Brushing someone's hair because no one else will.

We hold space not just for bodies -- but for dignity.

We see when someone hasn't had a visitor in weeks.
We notice the chipped nail polish and bring in remover from home.
We catch the silence that means someone has stopped feeling seen.

And we do what needs to be done.

Not because it's in the protocol.
But because it's in our bones.

Because sometimes the most sacred thing we can offer isn't a solution --

It's presence.

That day, brushing her hair reminded me why I became a nurse.
Not just to treat illness.
But to care for people.

To honor the pieces of them the world forgets to value.
And to remind them -- and sometimes myself -- that being human is enough.

Chapter

6

Do You Have a Minute?

It always starts the same way.
A quiet voice.
A glance toward the door.
A pause.
Then – "Do you have a minute?"

It's never just a minute.

It means:
I'm scared.
I need someone to see me.
I don't know how to say this to my family.
I don't know how to carry this alone anymore.

Sometimes it happens as I'm turning off the IV pump.
Other times, it's in the hallway -- one foot out the door, when I should already be in the next room.
But that question, "Do you have a minute?" -- it pulls me back. Because I know.
That minute matters.

There was a man once who kept pressing his call light for no reason.
When I'd go in, he'd say he was fine.
Then buzz again. Finally, I sat down and asked what was really going on. That's when he said it:
"Do you have a minute?"
He didn't need meds or vitals.
He needed to tell someone what he'd done.
Mistakes he'd never owned. People he'd never apologized to.
He wasn't asking me to fix it.
He just needed a witness.

Another time, a woman reached for my hand as I adjusted her IV. She looked right at me and said, "Do you think I'm dying?"
She didn't need comfort.
She needed honesty.
She needed me to stay long enough to say it without flinching.

Sometimes Do you have a minute? leads to a story.
Sometimes a confession.
Sometimes a goodbye in disguise.

One woman asked if I'd write down her passwords. Not because she was planning to die that day – but because she knew no one else would think of it until it was too late.

I've stood in stairwells listening to a patient describe how their husband never forgave them.
I've heard jokes that were really cries for help.
I've nodded quietly while someone told me about a child they gave up and never saw again.

These are the stories that never get documented.

They don't count toward outcomes or reimbursements.
But they count to us.

Because what people really want -- what they always want -- is presence.

Not answers. Not fixes. Just presence.
Someone willing to sit in the discomfort and not look away.

Sometimes what comes after "Do you have a minute?" changes you.
You carry it home.
You replay it in the car.
You think of it months later, folding laundry, wondering what became of them.

I've learned to say yes to those minutes.
Even when I'm tired.
Even when I'm behind.
Because those are the minutes that make this work human.

Do you have a minute?
It's not a question.

It's a quiet kind of trust.
A hand held out in the dark.
And the answer -- for as long as I can manage -- is yes.

Chapter

7

The Things That Still Trap Us

He had Parkinson's.
His movements were stiff, his body unreliable.
But his mind -- his mind was precise. Sharp. Intact.
You could feel it the moment you walked into the room.

He had been a prisoner of war in Vietnam.
And even though decades had passed, that experience never really left him.

Some kinds of trauma settle into the bones.
They shape the way a person breathes.
The way they move through space.
The way they sleep -- or don't.

I cared for him long enough that our relationship shifted.
He trusted me, slowly.
I'd bring my lunch into his room just to sit with him -- not because he needed anything urgently, but because I wanted to understand the man behind the chart.

One day, I noticed his bed hadn't been touched.
His blankets were still perfectly folded. His pillow undisturbed.

Instead, he was sleeping in a recliner, angled awkwardly, surrounded by chairs and equipment.

I asked gently, "Why don't you sleep in the bed?"

He paused.

Then he looked at me -- really looked -- and said, "They used to trap me in beds. Tie me down. Confine me."
He gestured to the hospital room. "This space reminds me of that. When I wake up and the bed's there -- I feel like I'm back."

He wasn't confused.
He wasn't exaggerating.
He was telling me what trauma still does, even now, even here -- in a place meant to heal.

I asked if we could try something.

We moved the furniture.
We cleared space.
We left the bed untouched, just as he wanted.

We gave him choice -- not just over where he slept, but over how he existed in a room that once would have felt like a cell.

The next day, I saw the difference.
He looked me in the eye.
His posture was more at ease.
He said, "Thank you."
And I knew exactly what he meant.

Because trauma doesn't end when the danger is over.
It lives on.
In layout.
In light.
In locked doors.

In unexpected beeping.

And nurses? We become architects of peace, in places where peace is hard to find.

We notice what doesn't make sense to anyone else -- and we listen until it does.

We ask, "How can we make this feel safer?"
Even if that means breaking the rules.
Even if it's not in the care plan.

Because some people never stop surviving.
And our job, sometimes, is to make surviving feel less lonely.

He wasn't the only one.
I've seen patients flinch when a curtain closes too fast.
I've seen women shut down when a male voice echoes through a hallway.
I've seen veterans tremble at the sound of boots on tile.
I've seen children panic at fluorescent lights.

Not all trauma is visible.
Not all traps are made of walls.

But when we notice -- when we adjust the space, or our voice, or the rhythm of the room -- something shifts.

Safety becomes possible.

And for people who've been through the unthinkable, possible is everything.

Chapter

8

Worn Thin

Theres a kind of tired that sleep doesnt touch.

It settles in your bones after too many years of holding grief in one hand and a chart in the other.
Its the fatigue that follows you home, that you try to shake off in the shower or drown out with a glass of wine or a scroll through your phone but it lingers.

Not because youre weak.
But because what you carry is heavy.
Nursing wears us thin.
Not just physically but emotionally, spiritually, soulfully.
And the worst part is how quietly it happens.
You show up for shift after shift.
You stay calm when others fall apart.
You keep your face soft when the news is bad.

You sit with dying people and hold the hands of their loved ones and then go warm up a cup of coffee like you didnt just witness the most sacred moment of someones life.

And you do it again tomorrow.

You dont even realize how thin youve become how scraped and stretched and silently aching until something small breaks you open.

The wrong song on the radio.
The way a patient says thank you.
A pair of shoes left by the door.

You find yourself crying in the car, in the bathroom, in the middle of folding laundry and you dont know which patient its really for.

Because its not just one.
Its all of them.
Its the father who coded.
The teenager who didnt wake up.

The grandmother who reminded you of your own.
The mother your age with the same diagnosis you keep worrying about for yourself.
Its the patients you couldnt save.
The ones you did but still wonder about.
The ones who looked at you like you were the only solid thing in their world and you smiled like you were fine.

Even when you werent.
Especially when you werent.
Theres a spiritual toll in pretending to be okay when your own world feels like its unraveling.
You show up to work and put your own pain in a box.
You dont talk about your divorce or your depression or your lost pregnancy.
You dont bring your grief or your fear into the room.
Because theres no space for it.
Because they need you to be strong.
Because how are you? isnt something you can answer honestly at a nurses station.
So you carry it.

You carry the pain youve seen and the pain you hide and you do it quietly.
Because thats what we do.
Were taught to hold space.
But no one teaches us how to refill it.
They talk about burnout like its a calendar issue.
Like you just need a weekend off or a better sleep schedule.
But its not your body thats breaking.

Its your spirit.

You start to question why you keep doing this.
You wonder if its worth it.
If you've made a mistake.
If there's something wrong with you for not being able to shake it off.
There's no CPT code for that.
No wellness seminar that touches it.
Because what were talking about isnt wellness.
Its survival.
And too many nurses are barely hanging on.
They smile.
They chart.
They manage a dozen things at once.
And then they go home and sit in their car in the driveway, too numb to move.
They scroll job postings.
They fantasize about quitting.
They whisper to themselves, I cant do this anymore.
Not because they dont love the work.
But because theyre empty.
And theyre ashamed of it.
Because nursing is supposed to be a calling, right?
Youre supposed to feel grateful.
Youre supposed to feel fulfilled.
So what do you do when it feels like its killing you?

When every shift chips away a little more of your softness, your hope, your belief in a world where people dont die alone and pain is always controlled and every patient has a family who shows up?

What do you do when the job you once felt called to now feels like a weight you cant set down?

You keep going.

Because its what we do.
But thats how we get worn thin.
It doesnt happen all at once.

It happens in the moments we dont grieve.
In the stories we dont tell.
In the trauma we normalize because weve seen worse.
We dont notice it until the pieces of ourselves we used to protect are gone.
The part that used to feel joy.
The part that used to believe we could make a difference.
The part that used to walk into work with a sense of purpose instead of dread.
I remember a day when I realized I hadnt laughed in weeks.
Not a real laugh.
Not the kind that shakes loose the dust in your chest and makes you feel human again.
And I thought: When did I become this person?

This tired.
This cynical.
This quietly hopeless.
And the answer wasnt in a specific shift.
It was in all of them.
All the nights I stayed late to call families.
All the codes.
All the can I talk to you for a minute? moments that turned into hours of emotional labor with no relief.

All the times I sat with patients and offered peace while silently begging the universe for my own.

We hold so much.

We hold stories no one else hears.

We hold the sobbing daughter and the guilt-ridden spouse and the quiet terror in a patients eyes.

We hold the weight of systems that fail and the guilt of not being able to fix whats broken.

And its beautiful.

But its brutal too.

Because holding all of that without a place to set it down will hollow you out.

We were never meant to carry it all alone.

And yet, we do.

Because the minute we set it down, someone else needs us.

And were the ones who say yes.

Even when our own hands are shaking.

Thats why the spiritual toll hits so hard.

Because its not just about what we see its about what it does to our sense of self.

To our faith in meaning.

To our belief that were making a difference.

We start to wonder if it matters.

If anyone notices.

If anyone would even know how much we gave not just our time and our labor, but the parts of ourselves we dont know how to get back.

Theres grief in that.

Real grief.

The kind that comes when you realize youve been pouring from a cup no one refills.

And its not fixed by a long weekend or a pizza party in the breakroom.

Its only fixed by telling the truth.

By saying: Im not okay.

By saying: This work is holy and its destroying me.

By saying: I need help.
We dont say that enough.
Were not allowed to.
But we should.
Because theres no shame in being human.
Theres no shame in being broken open by the things we witness.
Theres no shame in needing space to fall apart after holding everyone else together.

The shame is in pretending we dont feel it.
The shame is in systems that expect us to absorb the unthinkable and keep smiling.
The shame is in silence.
But were not silent anymore.
Not here.
Because here, we tell the truth.
We say that nursing is a spiritual experience one that will stretch you, shake you, sometimes shatter you.
We say that its okay to feel like youre losing parts of yourself.
We say that what you carry matters.
And that you matter.
Even if no one has told you lately.
Even if you feel invisible.
Even if all you did today was show up and survive.
Thats enough.
You are enough.
Even worn thin, you are sacred.

9

No Visitors Allowed

We used to whisper the words like a warning:
No visitors allowed.
It was the policy.
The protocol.
The shield that protected the hospital from infection and the rest of us from unraveling in front of each other.
But it became something more than that.
It became a mantra.
A line in the sand.
A reason for silence.

A weight we carried when we walked out of the hospital and into our homes homes that felt less like refuge and more like quarantine stations.

It was supposed to keep everyone safe.
But it left us shattered.
The early days of COVID were terrifying.
Not just because of the virus but because of the unknown.
We didnt know what we were walking into every shift.
We didnt know how bad it would get.
We didnt know if the gear we wore would protect us.
We didnt know if we were bringing death home with us on our scrubs.

And we were told not to ask too many questions.
Just show up.
Put the gear on.
Do the work.
Hold the iPad while a family says goodbye.
Tell the mother, the daughter, the son, No visitors allowed.
Then go home.

Alone.
Because thats what we did.
We isolated ourselves.
From our kids. Our spouses. Our parents. Our friends.
I remember driving home after those shifts hands red from sanitizer, chest heavy from the N95 mask still hanging from the rearview.
I'd change in the garage.
Put my shoes in a bin.
Walk through the house like a ghost, careful not to touch anything.
Careful not to breathe too close to anyone I loved.
I slept in the guest room for weeks.
Ate dinner alone.
Didnt let my children hug me.
Didnt let myself cry not until the water was running in the shower, and no one could hear.
And even then, I kept my sobs silent.
Because I didnt want to scare anyone.
I didnt want them to know how scared I was.
We were praised in public.
Hailed as heroes.
People banged pots and pans from their porches at 7pm.
But behind the closed doors of our homes, we were lonely.
Alienated.
Haunted.
We stopped talking about it with each other.
Stopped texting after shifts.
No one wanted to relive what wed seen.
The truth was too heavy.

We were watching people die alone.

Holding phones to their ears while their families sobbed from miles away.

Trying to comfort strangers with eyes full of panic and faces covered in PPE.

Trying to stay human when we couldnt show our own faces.

There were moments Id lean over a patient and wonder What if this is the moment I get it? What if I'm next?

I'd feel the sting of sweat inside my mask and think *Do I even have a fever? Or am I just terrified?*

There was no space for uncertainty.

We had to keep moving.

Keep charting.

Keep suctioning, bagging, flipping, medicating.

Keep saying Youre doing okay to people who werent.

Wed walk into COVID rooms over and over, and then wed walk out not into comfort, but into empty homes.

No one waiting with dinner.

No hugs.

No soft landing.

Because no one wanted to risk it.

We isolated to protect them.

But no one thought about what that meant for us.

How the absence of human contact eats away at your will.

How the silence in a house where no one touches you can feel louder than any monitor.

We were touch-deprived.

Soul-starved.

Exhausted not just physically, but spiritually from holding pain and then trying to disappear it by morning.

I remember watching my daughter play outside through the window and thinking, What if she loses me?

What if this is the shift that infects me?

What if this is the week I bring it home?

And I wouldve accepted it I really wouldve if it meant shed never have to be the one in the hospital bed with no one allowed in.

But I also remember thinking: Who takes care of us?

Who comes into our rooms when were breaking?

Who holds our hand while we say goodbye to our old lives, our old selves, the part of us that believed we could do this forever?

Because something died in us during that time.

A sense of safety.

A belief that hard work is enough.

A quiet hope that wed always be able to handle it.

We kept showing up.

But it took something.

And for many of us, that something hasnt come back.

Even now, we flinch when we hear a cough.

We carry the ghost of those shifts in the tension in our shoulders, the insomnia, the nightmares we dont talk about.

Some of us left the bedside.

Some of us stayed and learned to numb ourselves.

Some of us havent cried yet were still holding it all in.

Because we never got the time.

The space.

The chance to say: That was horrifying.

That was lonely.

That was traumatizing.

That changed me.

But we dont get time to process.

Because the world moved on.

No more pots and pans.

No more lawn signs.

No more grocery store priority lanes.

Just us with what we lived through.

Trying to keep going.

Still saying, No visitors allowed,

even when what we really mean is:

Please.

Dont leave us alone in this again.

Chapter

10

Ink and Gratitude

There are days we leave work feeling invisible.
Days we question if it all matters.
Not because we didnt give everything we had but because what we gave felt unseen.
Unacknowledged.
Absorbed into the void of another chaotic shift.

You clock out after twelve hours of caring, comforting, cleaning, advocating, and sometimes witnessing death and no one says a word.

Not even goodbye.
Thats what happens when the world gets used to you being the one who holds everything together.
You disappear into the role.
Into the task list.
Into the identity of someone who never needs anything in return.
But we do.

We need to be seen.
Not celebrated with fanfare or performative applause but seen as human.
And sometimes, all it takes is a thank you.

There was a patient once a woman in her 90s with a sharp tongue and soft eyes.
She wasnt in acute distress.
Just aging, inching closer to that quiet end that no one likes to talk about.
Her children lived across the country.
She had a few friends still hanging on.
But most days, it was just us.
Id help her to the chair in the morning.
Comb her hair.
Warm up her coffee.
Listen to the same stories the ones she repeated with increasing pauses between the words.

And I brought her dinner.
Not because I had to.
Not because it was in the care plan.
Because she told me one day that she missed real food.
So I made a plate.

At the end of my shift, I stopped by her room, handed it to her with a smile, and said, From my kitchen to yours.

She didnt cry.
She didnt make a big deal out of it.
But the next day, she told me it was the first time in weeks something had tasted like home.
That small comment carried me through days when I didnt think I could do it anymore.
Because most days, no one says anything.

Were not in it for the praise.
But praise reminds us that were not machines.
That someone noticed when we sat an extra minute at the bedside.
That someone remembered we were the ones holding the phone while they said goodbye.

That someone heard us say Youre not alone, and actually felt it.

Sometimes its a note.

Sometimes its a hug.

Sometimes its nothing more than a quiet, Thank you. I couldnt have gotten through that without you.

And it knocks the wind out of us.

Because were not used to being thanked.

Were used to being expected.

After a patient passes, the silence is loud.

You clean the body.

Wrap the belongings.

Call the family.

Document the time.

And then you move on.

But not really.

Because some patients stay with you.

The way they laughed.

The way they gripped your hand.

The way they told you they were scared, and you couldnt fix it, but you didn't leave.

There was one woman I'll never forget.

She'd been in our long-term care facility for months.

Her family was in Ohio.

We were in Colorado.

She had a decline not rapid, but steady.

And she was lonely.

So I used my own phone to FaceTime her daughters.

I sat with her while they talked.

Held the device when her hands trembled.

Stayed when she dozed off mid-call because they wanted to watch her sleep just for a minute.

I didnt do it for a thank-you.

But after she passed, they came back.

They found me in the hallway and handed me a gift: a frame with a poem she had written in calligraphy decades earlier.

She always said writing was her voice, her daughter whispered.

She'd want you to have this. You gave her back her voice.

I cried in the supply room.

Not because of the gift.

But because I felt remembered.

Seen.

Like who I was not just what I did mattered.

Small gifts hit hard because were not used to receiving anything.

We work holidays.

We miss birthdays.

We give pieces of ourselves to strangers and then try to rebuild whats left when we get home.

And most people never know.

We carry grief that doesnt have a name.

We carry stories we cant tell at dinner.

We carry moments that changed our lives but happened behind curtains with no witnesses.

So when someone says thank you;

When someone remembers your name;

When someone sends a card or frames a poem or brings you a coffee after a long shift;

It breaks something open.

In the best way.

Because it means they saw you.

Not as a nurse.

As you.

Theres a deep emotional wound in this profession: we give everything and are often left with nothing.

But then there are days when someone looks you in the eye and says, You mattered to me.

And suddenly, you can breathe again.

Thats what gratitude does.

It doesnt erase the trauma.

But it puts a light in the dark.

Sometimes it's not a patient.

Sometimes it's their family.

I remember a man who came back months after his wife passed.

He walked into our unit the same hallway where she took her last breath and stood in front of the nurses station with tears in his eyes.

I didn't know what to say before, he said. But now I just want to say thank you.

He handed us a tray of cookies and a note that read:

You were her angels. You helped me say goodbye with peace. I hope you never forget how important you are.

We didnt forget.

We never will.

Theres a kind of gratitude that lives beyond words.

It shows up in gestures.

In old photographs handed to us.

In cards with shaky handwriting that say, We see you.

And every nurse I know has a box somewhere.

A drawer.

A folder.

A little stash of cards, notes, scribbled thank-yous.

Because those are sacred.

Those are proof.

Proof that we were there.

That we mattered.

That we did something good in a world that too often forgets the quiet hands behind the healing.

Gratitude isnt the reason we do this work.

But it is the reason we survive it.

Because this work breaks you open.

And sometimes the only thing holding the pieces together is the memory of someone who looked at you and said, Thank you. You made this bearable.

Chapter

11

Hold Space for Us

We know how to hold space.
We do it without thinking.
When someone dies, we stay.
When someone grieves, we witness.
When someone breaks, we dont flinch.

We learn early in nursing school though no one says it outright that we are to be the emotional anchor. The still point in a storm. The place others collapse without worrying about who will catch them.

And we rise to it.
We show up.
We soften our voices.
We steady our hands.
We sit with people in the most broken moments of their lives and offer something that cant be charted: presence.

We know how to hold space.
But who holds it for us?
Theres no training for what happens after the shift.
No one prepares you for the silence of coming home after 12 hours of suffering.

No one tells you how to let go of the child you couldnt save.

No one warns you what it will feel like to see your own mothers eyes in a dying womans face and to still keep your voice calm and your hands clean and your charting complete.

Theres no debriefing.
No exhale.
No permission to feel.
Were expected to shake it off.

Move on.
Show up again tomorrow.

Strong.
But being strong starts to feel like a prison.
Because strength in this profession doesnt mean honesty it means hiding.
It means pushing through.
It means pretending youre fine so no one worries.
It means caring for everyone else while convincing yourself that you dont need care.
And its killing us.

I remember standing in the breakroom one night, staring at the vending machine like it might give me more than a soda. I wasnt hungry. I wasnt even tired. I was just done.

The patient Id been with for two weeks the one whose wife called every morning at 7 AM and every night at 9 had died.
I'd called her.
I'd walked her through his final moments.
I'd stayed with him so he wouldnt die alone.
And then I had four other patients to round on.
An admission.
A combative family member.
A medication error I caught before it caused harm.

A bed that needed to be changed.
A code in another unit.
By 3AM, I was empty.
And no one knew.
Because I smiled.
I joked.
I kept moving.
Thats what we do.
We know how to make others feel seen.

We ask, Do you want the lights on or off?
We pause to warm the blanket.
We notice when someone hasnt eaten.
We ask about the photo by the bedside.
But when was the last time someone noticed us?
Really noticed.
Not the nurse.
Not the worker.
Us.

The human underneath the badge.
The person grieving all the patients we never got to grieve.
The soul scraping together pieces of herself between shifts and hoping
no one sees the cracks.
Its not just that were exhausted.
Its that were lonely.
And not the kind of lonely thats fixed with a drink after work or a
group text.
Its the kind of loneliness that comes from giving everything and being
asked for more.
From listening to everyone and being heard by no one.
From holding space so often that we forget what it feels like to be held.
Sometimes we dont even know what were missing until someone gives
it to us.
A coworker who brings us a coffee without asking.
A patient who says, I see how hard youre working.

A friend who says, You dont have to be okay with me.

And we break.

Because we didnt realize how desperate we were to be seen.

One night, I stayed late to finish charting. Everyone else had gone home. The unit was dim, quiet. I was clicking boxes, writing notes I couldve written in my sleep. And I started crying.

Not loud.

Just soft, tired tears that came out of nowhere.

And I realized: no one knows what I carry.

No one knows that I was the one who held the teenagers hand as she coded.

No one knows that I still hear the voicemail from a daughter who never made it in time.

No one knows that I cant remember the last time I went a day without thinking of someone who died in my care.

We carry ghosts.

We carry guilt.

We carry grief that doesnt belong to us but stays anyway.

And we carry it in silence.

Because thats the unspoken rule: be strong, be steady, be selfless.

But its not sustainable.

We need space.

To feel.

To fall apart.

To say, This hurts, and not be told to toughen up.

To say, I cant do this alone anymore, and not be seen as weak.

We need someone to sit with us the way we sit with others.

Not to fix.

Not to problem-solve.

Just to witness.

To say, I see you.

Thats what it means to hold space.

And its what we deserve not just as nurses, but as people.

Sometimes we get glimpses.

A coworker pulls you aside and says, You okay?

A patient tells you, You remind me of my daughter.

A family member sends a card, and it says, You mattered to us.

And those moments they stay.

They become the rope we hold when were slipping.

They dont erase the trauma.

But they make it bearable.

Because someone saw us.

And chose to hold space for us even if only for a minute.

I wish we talked about this more.

I wish every shift came with a pause.

A circle of chairs.

A place where we could say, That was hard, and not be told to suck it up.

I wish managers asked how we were feeling not just what we were behind on.

I wish we had rituals for our grief.

I wish we lit candles.

I wish we named our dead.

I wish we stopped pretending that being a nurse means being invincible.

Because were not.

Were soft.

Were tired.

Were holy in our humanity and still somehow expected to keep giving from an empty well.

Thats not fair.

And its not okay.

To hold space means to allow to make room for what is.

We do that for others every day.

We say, You dont have to be okay.

We say, This is hard.

We say, I'm here.

But its time we heard those words ourselves.

Its time someone said them to us.

Its time we stopped expecting nurses to hold the weight of the world without offering a place to lay it down.

So if youre reading this if youre a nurse, a caregiver, a healer whos been holding space without anyone holding it for you I see you.

I see your tired eyes and your strong hands.
I see the way you hide your tears behind a busy shift.
I see the way you stay steady while breaking inside.
And Im holding space for you now.
You dont have to be strong today.
You just have to be real.
You just have to show up exactly as you are.
Thats enough.
You are enough.
And you deserve someone to hold space for you, too.

12

What I Hope You Remember

We see everything.
Thats the part people dont understand.
We see joy. Birth. Reunion. Recovery.

We see hope raw and bright when a patient stands up for the first time or a child opens their eyes or a family breathes again after the longest night of their life.

But we also see death.
We see pain that no one talks about in polite conversation.
We see people gasp for air, cry out in panic, look at us with eyes that say please dont let me die, even as the monitors flatline.
We see grief.
We see rage.
We see neglect.
We see miracles.
And we see all of it sometimes in the same shift, the same hallway, the same goddamn room.
We see it, we carry it, and then we go home like everyone else.
But we are not like everyone else.
I hope you remember that when we say were fine, it often means the opposite.

It means we havent had a moment to process the teenager who coded.
Or the grandmother who passed alone.
Or the young man who reminded us of someone we loved and lost.
It means were still carrying the voice of a wife who whispered goodbye over speakerphone.
Still thinking about the child who asked, Am I going to die?
Still wondering if we couldve done more.
We go from room to room, from trauma to tenderness, from CPR to discharge instructions and somehow were expected to be okay.
But were not always okay.
And that doesn't make us weak.
It makes us human.
I hope you remember that we dont leave it all at the hospital.
We try.
We wash our hands, wipe down our badges, scrub the memories off our scrubs.
But some things dont come off.
Some things come home with us in our bones, in our dreams, in the way we hesitate before answering *How was your day?*
We carry stories we cant share at the dinner table.
We carry faces we cant forget.
We carry moments that changed us in ways well never be able to explain.
We dont always cry about it.
Sometimes we just stare at the wall.
Or zone out during a movie.
Or flinch when a certain alarm sounds on TV.
Because its still in us.
And weve never had a safe place to set it down.
I hope you remember that nurses are not machines.
We are not just anything.
We are not replaceable parts in a system.
We are not robots with stethoscopes.
We are not immune to the trauma of what we see.
We are soft.
We are strong.
We are tired.

We are trained to manage chaos, but not always to heal from it.
We know how to hold space for you.
But no one ever taught us how to hold space for ourselves.
I hope you remember that every shift is a spiritual battlefield.
We witness the human condition in its rawest form.
We watch people lose everything.
We watch them gain it back.
We watch them fight.
We watch them give up.
We hear confessions, regrets, last words.
We listen when families yell at each other in grief.
We offer silence when no words will do.
And then we go to the next patient.
Because we have to.
Because someones waiting.
Because someone needs pain meds. Or wound care. Or help to the bathroom. Or to be held while they cry.
So we push it all down.
We say, You okay? with a soft hand on the shoulder.
We dont say, Im not.
I hope you remember that sometimes we cry in our cars.
We cry after nights that shouldnt have happened.
After codes that failed.
After watching someone die who reminded us too much of ourselves.
We cry from exhaustion.
From guilt.
From the weight of holding it all and pretending it doesnt crush us.
Sometimes we scream.
Sometimes we sit in silence, too numb for either.
We dont want pity.
We want permission.
To speak the truth.
To tell the stories.
To say, That was horrible and Im still not okay.
We want space to say:
That changed me.

That broke me.

That made me question everything.

We want space to say:

I need help too.

I hope you remember that we see the best and worst of humanity every single shift.

We see families fighting over DNR orders.

We see daughters singing lullabies to their dying fathers.

We see patients lie.

We see patients forgive.

We see racism.

We see grace.

We see the full, complex, beautiful, messy spectrum of what it means to be alive and to die.

And then we go back the next day and do it again.

Because we care.

Even when it costs us.

Even when it leaves scars no one sees.

What I hope you remember more than anything is that we need space too.

Not a wellness module.

Not a pizza party.

Not a pat on the back or a hashtag.

We need real space.

To speak.

To scream.

To rest.

To feel.

To be broken.

To be whole.

To be us without performing strength for a world that doesnt know what weve seen.

What I hope you remember is that when we say Im a nurse, its not a job title.

It's a vow.

To stand witness to what others cant bear.

To walk into rooms no one wants to enter.
To hold hands that are shaking.
To offer presence when there are no more answers.
And to keep showing up.
Even when no one is holding space for us.

CLOSING REFLECTION

This work will never leave me.
Not because I can't let it go --
But because it became part of who I am.

Every story.
Every silence.
Every whispered goodbye.
They live somewhere inside me now.

I used to think being a nurse meant knowing what to do.
Now I know it means being willing to stay --
Even when there are no answers.

We are more than caregivers.
We are witnesses.
We are translators of pain.
Holders of hope.
Bearers of truth in a world that often looks away.

People ask how we do it.
The truth is, sometimes we don't.
Sometimes we fall apart in the car.
Sometimes we cry in the bathroom between patients.
Sometimes we wonder if we can keep showing up.

But we do.
Not because we're unbreakable --
But because we are deeply breakable --
And still we choose to return.

That is the soul of nursing.

Not perfection.
Not martyrdom.
But the quiet decision, over and over, to stand in hard places with open
hands.

We show up because someone needs us.
We stay because it matters.
And we carry what others cannot --
Because at some point, someone did that for us.

So if you've read this far --
Thank you.
For bearing witness to us.

May we never forget the ones we cared for.
May we never forget each other.
And may someone, somewhere, hold space for you --
The way you've held space for the world.

www.ingramcontent.com/pod-product-compliance
Lightning Source LLC
Chambersburg PA
CBHW032215040426
42449CB00005B/604